10 Pov

Steps to Clear

Psoriasis

Based on 20 years experience ' Backed
by cutting-edge research into the human
microbiome

Lianne Campbell MSc

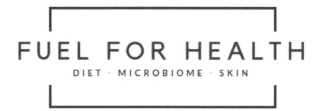

FUEL FOR HEALTH

DIET · MICROBIOME · SKIN

Disclaimer

This book does not provide medical advice. It is for information purposes only. Viewing this book, receipt of information contained in this book or transmission of information from this book does not constitute a physician–patient relationship. Do not disregard medical advice or delay seeking it. Fuel for Health and Lianne Campbell MSc assume no responsibility for the improper use of the information in this book.

Reviews of Lianne's first book *Healed*.

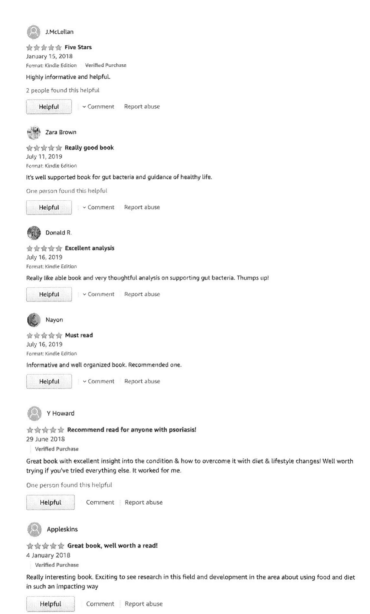

J.McLellan

★★★★★ **Five Stars**
January 15, 2018
Format: Kindle Edition   Verified Purchase

Highly informative and helpful.

2 people found this helpful

Helpful   ⌄ Comment   Report abuse

Zara Brown

★★★★★ **Really good book**
July 11, 2019
Format: Kindle Edition

It's well supported book for gut bacteria and guidance of healthy life.

One person found this helpful

Helpful   ⌄ Comment   Report abuse

Donald R.

★★★★★ **Excellent analysis**
July 16, 2019
Format: Kindle Edition

Really like able book and very thoughtful analysis on supporting gut bacteria. Thumps up!

Helpful   ⌄ Comment   Report abuse

Nayon

★★★★★ **Must read**
July 16, 2019
Format: Kindle Edition

Informative and well organized book. Recommended one.

Helpful   ⌄ Comment   Report abuse

Y Howard

★★★★★ **Recommend read for anyone with psoriasis!**
29 June 2018
   Verified Purchase

Great book with excellent insight into the condition & how to overcome it with diet & lifestyle changes! Well worth trying if you've tried everything else. It worked for me.

One person found this helpful

Helpful   Comment   Report abuse

Appleskins

★★★★★ **Great book, well worth a read!**
4 January 2018
   Verified Purchase

Really interesting book. Exciting to see research in this field and development in the area about using food and diet in such an impacting way

Helpful   Comment   Report abuse

Contents

"I have no special talent. I am only passionately curious."
Albert Einstein

HELLO

◆——— • ● ◆ ● • ———◆

Today is a good day.

Today is a good day because today is the first day of the rest of your life.

Whether you've had psoriasis for a long time, like I did (18 years), or you've recently been diagnosed, today is going to change things.

Whatever has happened in the past has happened: the days, the weeks, the years of topical treatments, UVB and biological medication; the many failed attempts to heal your skin; the perpetual loop of short-term remission through conventional treatments and the (possibly) years of depression and isolation – they are all behind you now…

This is the beginning.

This is the beginning of something new.

You might be conditioned into thinking that diet and lifestyle do not impact your skin, and it doesn't matter what you do or what you eat – your psoriasis will remain – but this is simply not true. You might have heard doctors, dermatologists, nutritionists and even your Auntie Jean (who may also have psoriasis) saying, "there is a lack of evidence that diet and lifestyle impacts psoriasis", and they would be 100% correct. There is a serious dearth of evidence relating to diet and lifestyle intervention for psoriasis because of the lack of research in this area. Founded in 1996, the British Skin Foundation has, according to their website, supported 400 research projects and awarded £16,000,000 in funding across all skin diseases. Can you guess how many research projects were about diet? One – a study in 2014 entitled, "The effect of nutritional status on clearance and remission of psoriasis following phototherapy".

This needs to change.

What does not exist is a powerful body of evidence to suggest that diet and lifestyle does not play a critical role in psoriasis. In fact, as research progresses, it is becoming more and more apparent that these factors play a huge role in the condition.

While research was being undertaken for this book, this study by Madden et al. was published: How lifestyle factors and their associated pathogenetic mechanisms impact psoriasis. The study states that,

"Lifestyle interventions are a promising treatment for psoriasis and its associated co-morbidities. However, gaps and inadequacies exist within the literature, e.g. methodology, absence of a unified scoring system, lack of controlled clinical data and lack of studies without simultaneous usage of biologics or alternative therapies."

Very few robust studies have been undertaken into diet and lifestyle interventions for psoriasis. Luckily for me, and for the 125 million people with psoriasis out there, a powerful body of research is emerging relating to the human microbiome (basically trillions of bacteria that populate every part of your body, internal and external) and "autoimmune" disease, which demonstrates that diet has a significant impact on you, your health and your skin.

During my study of psoriasis, spanning two decades, I became fascinated by this research. Your body hosts an ecosystem of single-celled organisms – imagine trillions of teeny, tiny chemists living in and on our bodies. From the microbes in our stomachs to the ones on our teeth, millions of these unique and diverse communities make their homes inside us and help our bodies function. Feeling itchy yet?

The gut is a hotbed of microbial action. Hippocrates called it when he said, "all disease begins in the gut", and, "let food be thy medicine and medicine be thy food" – we now know that the gut has a big impact on our health because of the 100 trillion bacteria living there. These tiny organisms play a major part in our health and our lives but have not been taken into consideration in our current medical system or food. You can read more about this in my first book, Healed.

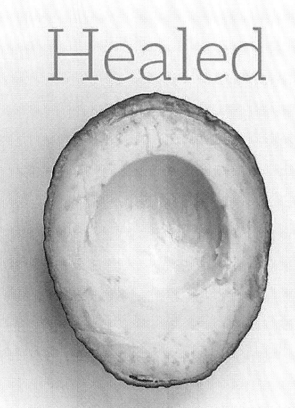

Lianne Campbell MSc

Healed

A science-based approach to support your gut bacteria and clear psoriasis.

PSORIASIS

◆———•●◆●•———◆

This paradigm shift in our understanding of the human body means that the basis of our entire healthcare system is on shaky foundations. A perfect example lies in the fact that, for the 18 years I had psoriasis, the condition was described as "autoimmune". Amy Poral now explains in her paper, _Reframing autoimmunity in an era of microbiome persistent pathogens autoantibodies molecular mimicry,_ that the theory of autoimmunity was developed at a time when the human body was regarded as largely sterile and antibodies in patients with chronic inflammatory disease could not be tied to persistent human pathogens. Amy concludes that, with our new understanding, the theory of autoimmunity needs to be revised to account for the human microbiome.

In 2016, the World Health Organisation (WHO) also published a Global report on psoriasis. The report stated that, "the etiology/aetiology of psoriasis remains unclear, although there is evidence for genetic predisposition. The role of the immune system in psoriasis causation is also a major topic of research. Although there is a suggestion that psoriasis could be an autoimmune disease, no autoantigen that could be responsible has been defined". The WHO added "yet" to the end of that sentence, but I have removed it as I believe this to be suggestive. So, for you and me, this means that nobody yet knows the root cause of psoriasis. This might come as a surprise or you might not find this surprising at all. However, what is surprising is the huge industry that has been built around the "unknown".

Despite the fact that we do not know the exact cause of the condition, the psoriasis pharmaceutical industry is set to be worth $21.4 billion by 2022. **$21.4 BILLION.**

2% to 3% of the total population has psoriasis – 125 million people worldwide – according to the World Psoriasis Day consortium. And, according to the National Psoriasis Foundation in America, patients with psoriasis incur annual healthcare costs that are significantly greater than those of the general population, amounting to $135 billion annually (2013 US $). The costs are thus hugely significant and lead to much dissatisfaction.

In the UK, we currently follow the NICE guidelines (see image 1 below) for psoriasis which are very NICE for pharmaceutical companies but not very NICE for patients. Patients end up in a perpetual loop of short-term treatments and topicals or extremely invasive and dangerous biologics and chemotherapy treatments while someone gets very wealthy.

I know this all too well as this is where I existed for 18 years.

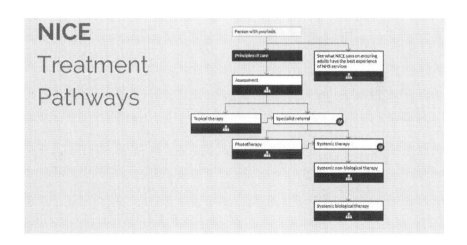

Image 1

Lack of understanding about the condition could explain why, despite treatment pathways and huge industry worth, psoriasis patients are dissatisfied and turning to alternative therapies. Patients frequently use complementary, alternative medicines for psoriasis when other therapies fail . This was certainly true for me. I tried every potion, lotion and crazy ideal going – everything from dousing myself in urine (my own) to a £3,000 trip to the Dead Sea. This is what happens when you are desperate.

What helped me, and eventually cleared my psoriasis, were other psoriasis patients, and I now hold them in the highest regard. They are, to date, the only experts in psoriasis I have encountered. Three people have had a significant impact on my skin healing – Matt Ludwig, Hanna Sillitoe and Nick Lamborghini. Thank you for your knowledge, your confidence to share, your strength to promote yourself and your message.

The fundamentals of this book are about using diet and lifestyle interventions to alter your overall biological state and modulate your microbiome. To date, conventional medicine can treat the symptoms of psoriasis, the skin lesions, and possibly even the immune response (with biologics), but they are yet to target the root cause (see image 2). This is a diagram I came up with to try and illustrate the point.

In the current structure, yes, topical steroids can help to suppress the skin lesions symptom of psoriasis, but the immune response remains. Yes, biologics and other immune suppressants can suppress the immune response (a pretty dangerous thing to do in my opinion) but, until you target the root cause, you will never really have a safe long-term treatment for psoriasis. What is also important to note here, is that the majority of research and investment in psoriasis (drugs and otherwise) have been focused at the middle and end of the disease pathway, not the start. This is starting to change.

PSORIASIS DISEASE PATHWAY

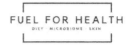

ROOT CAUSE	IMMUNE RESPONSE	SYMPTOM— SKIN LESIONS
(THAT CAUSES THE IMMUNE RESPONSE THAT CAUSES THE SYMPTOM)	(THAT CAUSES THE SYMPTOM)	(THE SYMPTOM—PSORIASIS)
	CURRENT TREATMENT	**CURRENT TREATMENT**
Epigenetic factors, disrupted gut bacteria (Dysbiosis, SIBO), molecular mimicry, opportunistic bacteria, intestinal permeability & immune reaction.	**Tablets, capsules & injections**— Non-biological medications—Methotrexate, Ciclosporin, Acitretin.	**Topical treatments**— Emollients, Steroids, Vitamin D analogue, Coal tar, Dithranol, Phototherapy— Ultraviolet B (UVB)
	Biological treatments— Etanercept, Adalimumab, Infliximab, Ustekinumab	**Phototherapy**—Psoralen plus ultraviolet A (PUVA), Combination light therapy.

DISEASE PATHWAY ⟶

Image 2

Another recent but critical change in psoriasis research is that the WHO has newly classified psoriasis a _non-communicable Disease (NCD)_: "non-communicable diseases (NCDs), also known as chronic diseases, tend to be of long duration and are the result of a combination of genetic, physiological, environmental and behaviours factors." Other NCDs include cardiovascular diseases (such as heart attacks and stroke), cancers, chronic respiratory diseases (for example, chronic obstructive pulmonary disease and asthma), as well as diabetes, Alzheimer's, osteoporosis and chronic lung disease.

It is believed that, "NCDs are caused 'to a substantial degree' by tobacco usage, alcohol abuse, poor eating habits and physical inactivity". That's not to say "healthy" people don't get psoriasis (or children or newborn babies) – it's just that all these factors significantly impact the human microbiome.

GUT BACTERIA

◆——— • ● ◆ ● • ——— ◆

S o, who am I, how did I come to have psoriasis and why am I writing this book?

Well, interestingly, as I trawled through my entire medical records in my late twenties, I discovered that my psoriasis started at age 16 after three rounds of broad-spectrum antibiotics, Amoxicillin, for tonsillitis. At that time, I was told the condition was genetic, autoimmune and incurable and I was put on a three-month waiting list to see a dermatologist.

When the appointment finally came around, the relief was overwhelming after three months of itchy, red, inflamed skin 24/7 on my elbows and knees. It was hell. If only I'd known that this was the tip of the iceberg.

At the appointment I had approximately five minutes with the specialist, who reviewed my skin, gave me some cream (which didn't work) and offered another appointment in three months' time. My heart was broken. I didn't realise then that this was the start of an 18-year cycle of dermatology appointments and short-term remission using conventional medicine. No wonder I became depressed.

All roads lead to Rome

In my years with psoriasis and my time at the Dead Sea, I met many people online and offline with stories to tell about their psoriasis, all different. I have spent my life trying to find a common thread stitching them all together. Here are some of the triggers I've heard about that created a shift in each of these individuals and started their psoriasis:

- Skiing accident
- Motorbike crash
- Excess stress – work, family, etc.
- Family death
- Illness
- Infection
- Cuts
- Alcohol abuse
- Change of external environment – moving to a new house
- Tonsillitis
- Antibiotics

According to Wang et al., "the gastrointestinal microbiota is influenced by a number of factors including genetics, host physiology (age of the host, disease, stress, etc.) and environmental factors such as living conditions and use of medications". It therefore seems that many of the things that impact the gut microbiota have an impact on psoriasis.

Stress appears to be a significant factor in microbiota changes and psoriasis onset. In the paper _Stress and psoriasis_, it was noted that, in a survey conducted by the international society of dermatology, in 31% to 88% of cases, patients reported stress as a trigger for their psoriasis. Another paper, _Psychosomatic paradigms in psoriasis: Psoriasis, stress and mental health_, published in 2013, stated that: "An outpatient skin clinic at King's College Hospital and the Psoriasis Association demonstrated that around 60% of those with psoriasis believe that stress/psychological factors are causal (in psoriasis)." A further case-control study reported high rates of stressful incidents having occurred before the onset of psoriasis in approximately 68% of adult patients.

So, what is the impact of stress on the gut/intestinal permeability? Well, according to the paper _Breaking down the barriers: the gut microbiome, intestinal permeability and stress-related psychiatric disorders_, "The emerging links between our gut microbiome and the central nervous system (CNS) are regarded as a paradigm shift in neuroscience with possible implications for not only understanding the pathophysiology of stress-related psychiatric disorders, but also their treatment." The paper goes on to explain that "the concept that a 'leaky gut' may facilitate communication between the microbiota and these key signalling pathways has gained traction. Deficits in intestinal permeability may underpin the chronic low-grade inflammation observed in disorders such as depression and the gut microbiome play a critical role in regulating intestinal permeability" (see figure 1).

Some really amazing work is happening in the area of the gut–brain connection, including an excellent book, The Psychobiotic Revolution.

Studies have now established that gut bacteria play a central role in

16

host homoeostasis and immune response, specifically in Th17 cells, which have been implicated in the development of psoriasis and other autoimmune diseases. The most recent paper published last year on this subject, The gut microbiome as a major regulator of the gut–skin axis, concluded that, "through complex immune mechanisms, the influence of the gut microbiome extends to involve distant organ systems including the skin. With intentional modulation of the microbiome, probiotics, prebiotics, and synbiotics have proven beneficial in the prevention and/or treatment of inflammatory skin diseases including acne vulgaris, AD, and psoriasis".

A possible genetic pre-disposition to the condition might exist. However, as previously mentioned, there is no test for psoriasis and researchers still aren't clear on the precise details of psoriasis-associated genetic links. The condition could manifest itself because of a "switching on" of the genes, known as epigenetics. Epigenetics is the study of heritable changes in gene function that do not involve changes in the DNA sequence, and these epigenetic factors (that "switch" on the gene) are often factors you control:

- Diet
- Lifestyle
- Excess stress
- Trauma
- Smoking
- Alcohol
- Bad diet
- Recreational drugs
- Pharmaceutical drugs
- Tonsillitis (broad-spectrum antibiotics – Amoxicillin)

This diagram from Five Seasons Medical is also useful in helping illustrate the complexities of this "autoimmune" disease. These external factors can all, to varying degrees, alter our genes through interplay with our microbiome.

When I finally reached the end of my tether with conventional options, I decided to go all in. My psoriasis was bad, and I was reading more and more online about diet and lifestyle intervention – it must be worth a shot. I had tried various diets for a month or two in the past but nothing had worked. I decided to go all in, 100%, with everything.

Before I embarked on diet and lifestyle changes, I tested my gut bacteria, and the results showed low diversity, low levels of probiotics and low-level Akkermansia (compared to the selected sample), which helps to manage inflammation. What is interesting is that in this recent study, The Akkermansia muciniphila is a gut microbiota signature in psoriasis, it was noted that:

"… the abundance of Akkermansia muciniphila was significantly reduced in patients with psoriasis. A. muciniphila is believed to have an important function in the pathogenesis of IBD and obesity; therefore, A. muciniphila, which is an indicator of health status, may be a key node for psoriasis as well as IBD and obesity. Taken together, our study identified that gut microbiota signature and function are significantly altered in the gut of patients with psoriasis, which provides a novel angle to understanding the pathogenesis of psoriasis."

You can see my gut bacteria profile and Akkermansia before and after diet changes, and before and after my psoriasis cleared.

Before:

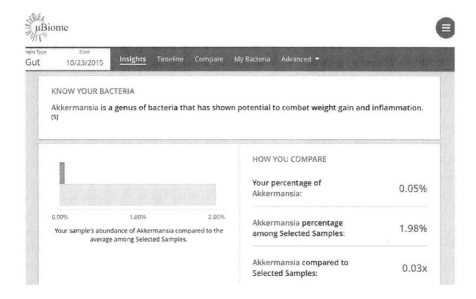

Image 3

After:

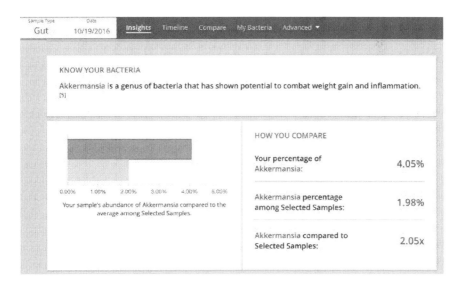

Image 4

DISRUPTION IN GUT BACTERIA

◆———— • ● ◆ ● • ————◆

What is becoming apparent is the impact of these epigenetic factors on gut bacteria and digestion. We are now beginning to know a lot more about the impact of gut bacteria on our health, including the following areas:

- Dysbiosis – microbial imbalance in the gut (can be Small Intestinal Bacterial Overgrowth (SIBO)).

- SIBO

    ◆ Overgrowth of yeast and other fungus and bad bacteria, including toxins produced by fungus and bacteria.

- Leaky and permeable gut – permeability in the gut lining. Gut dysbiosis leads to changes in the lining of the bowel that can increase the permeability of the intestine.

- Inflammation.

Harmful bacteria are the main cause of leaky gut syndrome. However, we know that alcohol, gluten, dairy, food additives, antibiotics and pesticides can contribute to issues with gut bacteria and also damage the gut wall. These substances can cause more issues when bacteria in the gut are compromised. When damaging particles make their way into the bloodstream, the body looks for the fastest way to remove them. The skin is often the quickest option. This triggers an immune reaction which can cause redness, swelling and itchiness.

I read a recent study entitled, <u>Leaky gut as a danger signal for autoimmune diseases</u>, which stated that, "translocation of intestinal microbial components into the bloodstream caused by dysbiosis-induced leaky gut can increase the risk of autoimmune diseases". This basically states that the movement of gut bacteria (or opportunistic fungus in the gut which have enjoyed a flourishing environment because of low acid production caused by triggers such as stress, trauma and antibiotics) into the bloodstream is caused by imbalances in the gut resulting in permeability. These particles are then free to be transported through the bloodstream and cause havoc in the body.

Here is a good visual explanation of <u>Leaky gut from Dr Axe</u>. Leaky gut and mycobiome (for example, candida) have long been considered as quackery or pseudo-science as there wasn't evidence to back them up. If you fancy an interesting read, check out the NHS take on "Leaky gut syndrome".

Now, however, it appears that, with microbiome sequencing and the focus on the gut, evidence is catching up with theory. There are now 14,778 items on PubMed on "intestinal permeability" and 342 items on the term "leaky gut", with the most significant number appearing in the last few years:

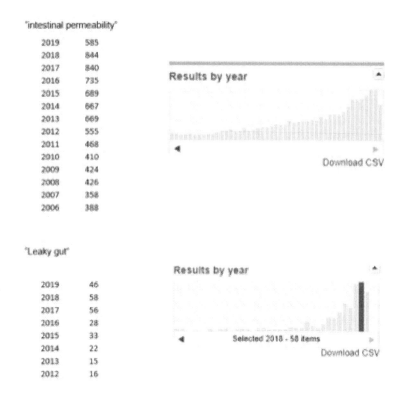

"intestinal permeability"

Year	Value
2019	585
2018	844
2017	840
2016	735
2015	689
2014	667
2013	669
2012	555
2011	468
2010	410
2009	424
2008	426
2007	358
2006	388

Results by year

Download CSV

"Leaky gut"

Year	Value
2019	46
2018	58
2017	56
2016	28
2015	33
2014	22
2013	15
2012	16

Results by year

Selected 2018 - 58 items

Download CSV

Regardless of how your psoriasis came about, I believe that it can be cleared by getting to its root cause and supporting your return to good health through diet and lifestyle intervention.

THE TIME IS NOW

◆──────•●◆●•──────◆

This book is short and sweet – no messing, no fluffy chat, no pretty pictures (ok, there might be one or two pretty pictures), no time wasting, because you have some serious healing to do and I don't want you to delay it. You have waited long enough.

Over the years I have seen every psoriasis specialist, from doctors to dermatologists to dieticians and aromatherapists. I have tried every lotion and potion and "miracle cure" and travelled the world searching for relief from this distressing, often isolating, and all-consuming condition. My pain is your gain.

In this book I lay down the most relevant and critical information if you need to heal psoriasis, and I do so with more than 20 years of experience and research. I have tried and failed, and tried and failed, and tried and failed again, to heal psoriasis (on a continual loop for 18 years) until I tried, and I succeeded.

In my lifetime I've read two degrees and completed my MSc with a distinction and a court medal. However, what I know from these pales in comparison to what I know about psoriasis. There may be some leaps in this book which the more scientific reader might struggle to make, but remember that I make these based on experience and not blind faith. Nothing in this book is high risk. There has been a lot of scaremongering and talk of "food shaming" amongst dieticians, with registered nutritionists recently telling you to "eat that cake/junk food". I appreciate their standpoints but, seriously, we don't really need anyone else advertising cake/junk food. It is important to note that there is nothing extreme here, just good advice founded on solid research and experience.

From my 18 years with psoriasis – living with it, reading about it and thinking about it, and my five years clear of psoriasis – writing and research the topic – I have pulled together the ten most powerful steps you can take to start clearing your psoriasis today.

Let's go!

STEP 1

MINDSET

◆——— • ● ◆ ● • ———◆

Before you embark on any changes in your life, your head must be in the game. You must wholeheartedly believe that your approach will work, despite a lack of success in the past, and you have to commit to this. This is your life – don't wake up another day with a negative attitude, don't waste another hour wishing or hoping or searching for a miracle. Change things now.

This was a game changer for me. When I finally healed my psoriasis completely after 18 years, it was a result of my wholehearted commitment with mind, body and soul. Everything lined up.

Despite the current medical approach to health (which breaks things up and segregates sections of your body), your body is connected – all of it. Your mind is therefore connected to your body, not in a spiritual/alternative way but in a scientifically factual and actual physiological way. Your mind and body therefore need to get in line for things to change.

I guess I am a very fortunate individual and have always had a growth mindset – even when I was diagnosed with psoriasis and lived with it for 18 years, I was always trying, always reading, always hoping that things would change, that life would improve and I would wear … shorts. It's a small wish, but when you have spent 18 months in Australia in 40-degree heat wearing trousers and long-sleeved tops every day, your personal goals shift dramatically. Wearing shorts and a t-shirt comfortably in public became a lifelong ambition for me.

I'd tried gluten-free diets and dairy-free diets and abstained from alcohol and nothing worked. In fact, on several occasions, things got worse (more on this later). I would plummet into depression repeatedly and had to dust myself off, pick myself up and get right back to it. I think it's known as falling forward – the belief that there is no failing, only learning; something to remember and embrace throughout this process.

Everyone is different and motivated by different things and there will be a few ups and downs along the way, but here are a few things that motivated me.

STEP 1 – POSITIVE ACTIONS

Reading or audiobooks

There are many good books on healing psoriasis from the root cause that I would recommend as worth a read while you are embarking on this new approach. Here are the ones that have had the greatest impact on me:

- Healing Psoriasis
- The Keystone Approach
- Healed (obviously)
- 10% Human
- The Microbiome Solution
- Radiant

Your mind can create a positive healing environment, setting all the wheels in motion for a huge turning point in your life, or create a loop of negativity and obsession that will keep you stuck and sick. There are a number of great books on the power of your mind to impact your body. Here are some of my favourites:

- The Source
- You Are the Placebo
- Biology of Belief

Psoriasis & microbiome research

Research is being shared daily about the impact of the microbiome and health. I would love to share all the key research relating to psoriasis. I have collated in excess of 80 papers relating to gut bacteria and diet and lifestyle intervention in psoriasis. To access this information, just sign up to my website on the home page www.fuelforhealth.co.uk with "psoriasis research" as the title.

Finding a tribe

Online or in life, having support can be critical to success. A couple of online tribes that worked well for me were **Psoriasis Healing Warriors** and **One Year No Beer**, both on Facebook.

STEP 2
INCREASE WATER INTAKE

◆———•●◆●•———◆

Increasing water intake is a simple but crucial step. Water is a critical part of healing your skin – water is a powerful tool to rid your body of waste through urination, perspiration and bowel movements (Centres for Disease Control and Prevention). Drinking more water not only helps to hydrate and clear you out, it also helps to keep your skin supple.

Lemon water

Drinking lemon or lime water daily was a fundamental part of clearing my psoriasis in the long term. I only did this for three months. I drank up to two litres of water per day – one with a whole lemon or lime and one made up of just water. I learned about this from Matt Ludwig and the other 15,000 psoriasis patients in the Psoriasis Healing Warriors group on Facebook, but I read the research on lemon water and it was fascinating.

Lemon water supports digestion (bile) and has a large spectrum of biological activity, including anti-bacterial, anti-fungal, anti-diabetic, anti-cancer and anti-viral activities. We know from research that *Long-term Western diet intake leads to dysregulated bile acid signalling and dermatitis with Th2 and Th17 pathway features in mice*. It would be interesting to see some studies on this in humans.

Lemon also contains flavonoids, which can function directly as antioxidants to savage free radicals in the body. Lemon supports digestion, which is much needed as you repair your gut and re-engineer your gut bacteria. Water also helps to flush out toxins. In addition, lemons promote the growth of gram-negative bacteria in our gut. Vitamin C in lemons and limes is a potent antioxidant that can help to lower inflammation in the gut. Lemons also contain pectin which is a prebiotic for gut bacteria and may help to promote growth of a healthy microbiome.

The 2018 study *Is psoriasis a bowel disease? Successful treatment with bile acids and bioflavonoids suggests it is* states:

"Bacterial peptidoglycans absorbed from the gut have direct toxic effects on the liver and skin." The study also argues that their absorption, as well as endotoxin absorption, needs to be eradicated to successfully treat psoriasis. They conclude that, "bioflavonoids, such as quercetin and citrus bioflavonoids, prevent this absorption".

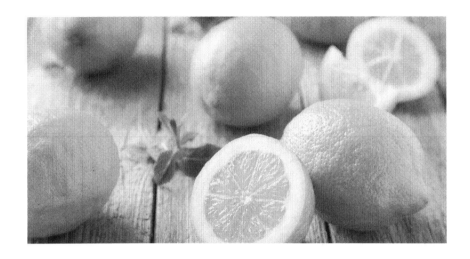

STEP 2 – POSITIVE ACTIONS

- Invest in a large BPA-free water bottle, keep in sight at work/ at home.

- Always order water when you are out, especially if you are drinking alcohol or sugary drinks.

- Set an alarm at work or at home every hour to make sure you are drinking; you can also incorporate it into a habit such as going to the printer or the toilet at work.

- As discussed above, it is important to drink lemon water, but you can also add cucumber or lime to make the water more appealing.

- When making lemon water there are some hacks – you can juice it in advance and add it to water throughout the week or freeze cubes of juiced lemon water and add it to your water.

- Drink water in herbal tea.

STEP 3

SALT BATHS & OILS

◆——— • ● ◆ ● • ———◆

One of the most powerful tools for clearing your skin is water and salts (magnesium). Part of a quick recovery from psoriasis is regular salt baths to increase your magnesium levels and bypass the digestive system. As with alkaline and mineral-rich diets, we are trying to flood the body with these health-giving minerals and alter the environment in the body for a healthy microbial balance. One of the quickest and easiest ways to do this is through bathing.

Salt bathing flooding the body with vital minerals - magnesium, sulfur, iodine, sodium, calcium, potassium, bromine - lacking in psoriasis patients due to Dysbiosis or Small Intestinal Bacterial Overgrowth

An increase in intracellular magnesium, which is required for the function of many enzyme systems, is another added benefit of the magnesium baths. Available magnesium, which is required to activate vitamin D, results in numerous added benefits in the vitamin D apocrine/exocrine systems. Vitamin D has a long connection with psoriasis as you may know from topical applications or UVB therapy. More about this in Step 10.

A study by Birmingham University concluded that bathing in Epsom salts is a safe and easy way to increase sulphate and magnesium levels in the body (report on absorption of magnesium sulphate (Epsom salts) across the skin). This is also a great article on exploring the: connection between psoriasis and magnesium deficiency? This talks about how bathing bypasses the digestive system and current state of gut microbiota to increase magnesium absorption.

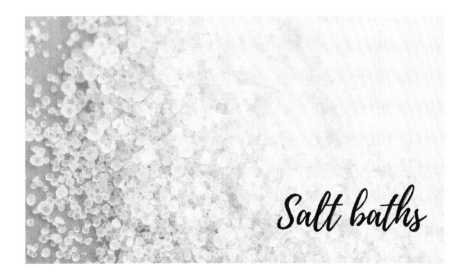

Salt baths

Essential oils

As part of your regular baths I would include drops of essential oil. Just put in what you can tolerate – don't overdo it as it might sting, but try and build up the amount you can tolerate each time you have a bath.

Various essential oils are proven to be excellent anti-bacterial agents. The key ones I would focus on/rotate are as follows:

- Tea tree

- Rosemary

- Eucalyptus

- Lavender

- Camomile

- Oregano (be very careful with this)

Here are some others and some more information – <u>Antibacterial essential oils: the top 10 choices for bacterial infections</u>

STEP 3 – POSITIVE ACTIONS

- I would recommend Epsom salts or Dead Sea salt baths every three days initially until you start seeing a difference in your skin. I would be generous with the salts – two cups minimum and sit in it for a minimum of 30 minutes, longer if you can.

- Include six to eight drops of essential oil in your bath where possible.

- I would try to keep this up (at least one or two baths a week) for at least three months.

- Enjoy!

STEP 4
EAT REAL FOOD

◆———— • ● ◆ ● • ————◆

"Put plants first" is a simple mantra when looking for a powerful way to change your eating and clear psoriasis. Plant-based eating has a big following now and rightly so – huge benefits arise from green plants and eating the rainbow for you and your gut bacteria. I would recommend upping the vegetables you enjoy (avoiding nightshades) and adding in leafy greens where possible.

I would highly recommend following the Harvard Healthy Eating Plate (see image 5 below). More information can be found on their website and the only caveat I would add to it for psoriasis is to avoid gluten. More on this in step 7 on removing inflammatories.

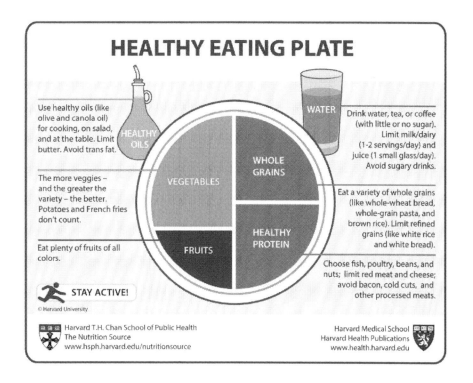

HEALTHY EATING PLATE

Use healthy oils (like olive and canola oil) for cooking, on salad, and at the table. Limit butter. Avoid trans fat.

HEALTHY OILS

The more veggies – and the greater the variety – the better. Potatoes and French fries don't count.

VEGETABLES

Eat plenty of fruits of all colors.

FRUITS

WHOLE GRAINS

HEALTHY PROTEIN

WATER

Drink water, tea, or coffee (with little or no sugar). Limit milk/dairy (1-2 servings/day) and juice (1 small glass/day). Avoid sugary drinks.

Eat a variety of whole grains (like whole-wheat bread, whole-grain pasta, and brown rice). Limit refined grains (like white rice and white bread).

Choose fish, poultry, beans, and nuts; limit red meat and cheese; avoid bacon, cold cuts, and other processed meats.

STAY ACTIVE!

© Harvard University

Harvard T.H. Chan School of Public Health
The Nutrition Source
www.hsph.harvard.edu/nutritionsource

Harvard Medical School
Harvard Health Publications
www.health.harvard.edu

Image 5

Many people promote the benefits of green drinks and smoothies for psoriasis and I would absolutely recommend these for quicker results. However, I didn't do a huge amount of this for my skin – I focused more on quick wins in terms of flooding my system with minerals, incorporating foods such as wheatgrass and lots of cucumber.

Drinks made from green vegetables and powdered grasses are loaded with apparent mineral-rich foods and help to support the body's natural state. When you juice, you can also lose a lot of the fibre needed by the gut bacteria, so ensure that you eat a lot of plant-based food too. Green juices and smoothies are great and there are lots of recipes out there that are low in fruit and sugar. I do recommend these, but you can clear psoriasis without green juices and smoothies if it's not your thing.

This diagram by Edward Ishiguro, Natasha Haskey and Kristina Campbell, which can be found in Gut Microbiota interactive effects on nutrition and health, highlights the dietary changes currently recommended in science for maintaining a health-associated microbiota.

It highlights fruit and vegetables, olive and flaxseed oil, nuts and seeds, prebiotics, resistant starches such as less ripe bananas and pulses, and fermented foods with live active cultures.

It also highlights dietary components that potentially modulate the microbiota in a detrimental way – red meat, omega-6 fats, a "Western diet", refined carbohydrates and processed foods.

This review on How lifestyle factors and their associated pathogenetic mechanisms impact psoriasis states that:

"Poor nutrition and low Omega 3 fatty acid intake, likely combined with fat malabsorption caused by gut dysbiosis and systemic inflammation, are associated with psoriasis. The data strongly suggest that improvements to disease severity can be made through dietary and lifestyle interventions and increased physical activity. Less conclusive, although worthy of mention, is the beneficial effect of bile acid supplementation."

Psoriasis diet list

Vegetables	Consume lots of vegetables, especially greens such as cucumber, celery, avocado, kale and broccoli, but also sweet potato, parsnip, butternut squash or anything in season. Eat raw or steamed where possible. I ate half a cucumber every day for two to three months.
Fermented foods	Fermented foods are packed with probiotics (good bacteria) such as sauerkraut, kimchi and kombucha. Yoghurt and kefir are also good sources of probiotics if you can tolerate them (dairy), although I would suggest sticking to non-dairy fermented foods for the first three months.
Nuts and seeds	Don't overdo these but take a selection of nuts and seeds regularly. These can be added to salads, stir fries and homemade cereals made with quinoa.
Plant proteins, meat and fish	It is important to ensure that you obtain as much food as you can to support your body. You can eat beans and lentils. I am intolerant to lentils so mainly ate white meats such as turkey, chicken and fish.

Carbohy-drates	I ate quinoa and white rice during the initial three months. I would have eaten brown rice and, if you can digest it, great, but I couldn't. Oats are another carbohydrate which are potentially good if you can tolerate them, but, again, I couldn't. I tried gluten-free oats too and these seemed to work for me.
Herbs and spices (avoid paprika and chilli)	These are great to add flavour to your food; it is also worth including apple cider vinegar where possible.
Drinks	These include water, green drinks/herbal teas and milk substitutes For ideas and recipes, follow @health-fuel on Twitter and @fuel_for_health on Instagram.

Diet research & surveys

Although there is a fundamental lack of research into diet and life-style intervention for psoriasis, the research that has been under-taken is very positive. When gut microbiota is disturbed, this can, as well as creating gut permeability, create issues with digestion of certain food. For me this certainly happened with dairy and gluten, but other things mentioned in many psoriasis diet books and refer-enced in the National Psoriasis Foundation survey are alcohol (which we will talk about later), gluten and nightshade food. I would avoid all of these, at least in the first three months, while clearing psoriasis.

This was an interesting study on Pagano/Edgar Cayce treatment: **Medical nutrition therapy as a potential complementary treatment for psoriasis – five case reports.** The five psoriasis cases, ranging from mild to severe at the study onset, improved on all measured outcomes over a six-month period:

"The five psoriasis cases, ranging from mild to severe at the study onset, improved on all measured outcomes over a six-month period when measured by the Psoriasis Area and Severity Index (PASI) (average pre- and post-test scores were 18.2 and 8.7, respectively), the Psoriasis Severity Scale (PSS) (average pre- and post-test scores were 14.6 and 5.4, respectively), and the lactulose/mannitol test of intestinal permeability (average pre- and post-test scores were 0.066 to 0.026, respectively). These results suggest a dietary regimen based on Edgar Cayce's readings may be an effective medical nutrition therapy for the complementary treatment of psoriasis; however, further research is warranted to confirm these results."

I contacted the person who led this study and they were told that no further funding was available to undertake a larger study or RCT.

In 2017, the NPF also surveyed 1,206 psoriasis sufferers to explore the effects of diet and lifestyle intervention. According to the NPF, the survey was conducted because psoriasis patients demonstrate a high interest in the role of diet in their skin condition:

"86% percent of respondents reported use of a dietary modification. The percentage of patients reporting skin improvement was greatest after reducing alcohol (53.8%), gluten (53.4%), nightshades (52.1%), and after adding fish oil/omega-3 (44.6%), vegetables (42.5%), and oral vitamin D (41%). Specific diets with the most patients reporting a favourable skin response were Pagano (72.2%), vegan (70%), and Palaeolithic (68.9%). Additionally, 41.8% of psoriasis respondents reported that a motivation for attempting dietary changes was to improve overall health." (see image 6)

PSORIASIS DIET & LIFESTYLE INTERVENTION

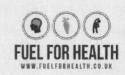

FUEL FOR HEALTH
WWW.FUELFORHEALTH.CO.UK

Results from the National
Psoriasis Foundation
Survey 2017

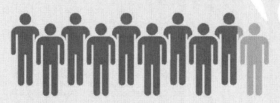

86%
OF RESPONDENTS
REPORTED USE OF
A **DIETARY**
MODIFICATION

THE PERCENTAGE OF PATIENTS REPORTING
SKIN IMPROVEMENT WAS GREATEST AFTER:

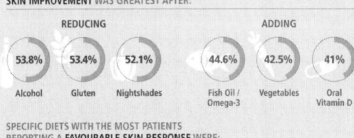

REDUCING			ADDING		
53.8%	53.4%	52.1%	44.6%	42.5%	41%
Alcohol	Gluten	Nightshades	Fish Oil / Omega-3	Vegetables	Oral Vitamin D

SPECIFIC DIETS WITH THE MOST PATIENTS
REPORTING A **FAVOURABLE SKIN RESPONSE** WERE:

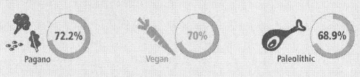

72.2%	70%	68.9%
Pagano	Vegan	Paleolithic

A TOTAL OF **1206 PSORIASIS PATIENTS** RESPONDED TO THE SURVEY

Image 6

STEP 4 – POSITIVE ACTIONS

- Follow the Harvard Healthy Eating Plate (minus nightshades and gluten). I would even recommend their six week course.

- Focus on the diet components that support gut bacteria.

- Keep it simple – eat healthy foods you can prepare, and that you like.

- Focus on what you are adding in, not what you are subtracting.

- Stop and relax when eating and, ideally, over-chew your food.

- Eat regularly – don't let your blood sugar levels drop as this can cause stress on the body, and stress can impact your psoriasis.

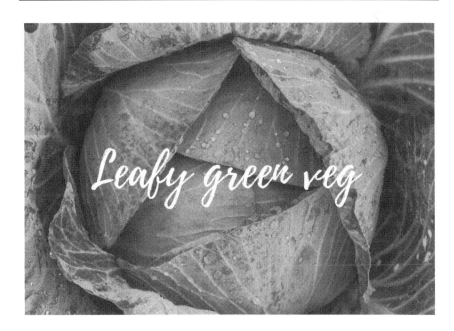

STEP 5
PREBIOTICS & PROBIOTICS

◆──── • ● ◆ ● • ────◆

Prebiotics and probiotics are an important part of gut recovery. To be honest, I am not a fan of taking supplements or popping pills, but a few worked for me. There is a lot of chat in the psoriasis community now about probiotics. This is about repopulating the gut with healthy bacteria. You can do this with fermented foods such as kimchi, kefir, kombucha or sauerkraut, or you can take a supplement. Expert advice on taking probiotics from Tim Spector (the Diet Myth guy) begins with fermented food. If you take a probiotic supplement, make sure it contains millions and make sure it's fresh/in date and that it comes from a reputable brand.

DDS – 1 Strain

Rightly or wrongly, there is lots of chat about DDS – 1 Strain in the psoriasis community and I have to say that, based on this, with no scientific evidence, this is what I took. However, I didn't eat a lot of probiotics and still don't, and this is evident in my test results. My probiotics were incredibly low compared to the general population (see image 7).

According to probiotic people, DDS – 1 Strain is associated with dairy digestion, supporting lactose intolerance and producing enzymes such as lactase, which makes sense for me, being lactose intolerant. I have also noticed the biggest reaction with dairy for my skin.

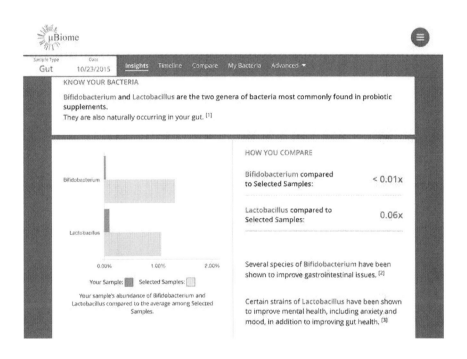

Image 7

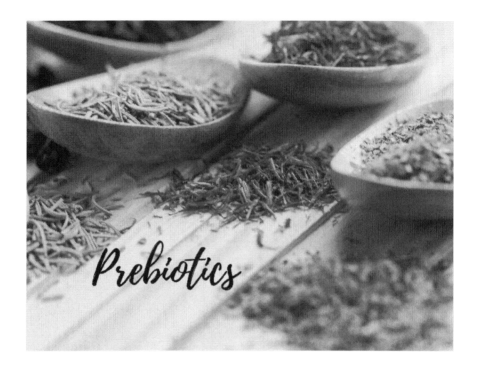

Prebiotics

Healing Psoriasis – Dr Pagano & Edgar Cayce

One of the first books I ever read about diet and psoriasis was *Healing Psoriasis* by Dr John Pagano, based on the work of Edgar Cayce. Pagano and Cayce are the OG of the psoriasis diet world and their arguments form the basis of many of the books and online protocols people use today. Interestingly, Edgar Cayce was a psychic, which is why, amongst other reasons, scientists, doctors and dermatologists are sceptical about his work. However, both Edgar Cayce and Dr Pagano suggested **psyllium husk** and **slippery elm** in their healing diets, which, given the lack of research into the gut microbiome at the time, is actually incredible as they are both prebiotics.

As mentioned earlier, 72.2% of the patients surveyed by the NPF who had tried diets reported full clearance or improvement with the Pagano diet. I tried to get in touch with Dr John Pagano but, unfortunately, he is no longer with us. I find this quite sad given his significant and important input into diet intervention for psoriasis.

Psyllium husk

Psyllium husk (Planta Ova) is a prebiotic, which means that it contains indigestible fibre, essentially creating food for our gut bacteria. These articles and studies are worth reading for more information:

♦ **The interplay between fibre and the intestinal microbiome in the inflammatory response**

♦ **Cytokine changes in gastric and colonic epithelial cell in response to Planta Ovata extract** – it decreased pro-inflammatory reaction from both cell lines stimulated by bacteria.

Slippery elm

Slippery elm contains mucilage, which helps to stimulate the production of mucus, a component of the gastrointestinal tract's protective lining. Slippery elm is also a prebiotic which is fermented by colonies of bacteria and helps to alter the composition of the microbiome

Triphala

This prebiotic is not part of the *Healing Psoriasis* protocol, but one I have come to learn about and admire through my research. It is an ancient ayurvedic medicine. According to research, "polyphenols in Triphala modulate the human gut microbiome and thereby promote the growth of beneficial Bifidobacteria and Lactobacillus while inhibiting the growth of undesirable gut microbes." The bioactivity of Triphala is stimulated by gut bacteria to generate a variety of anti-inflammatory compounds.

Coconut oil

Another interesting substance for consideration is coconut oil. Although not a prebiotic as such, coconut oil can kill harmful micro-organisms. 50% of the fatty acids in coconut oil are made up of the 12-carbon lauric acid. When lauric acid is digested, it forms a substance called monolaurin. Lauric acid and monolaurin can both kill harmful pathogens such as bacteria, viruses and fungi, and in fact have been shown to help kill the bacteria Staphylococcus aureus and the yeast Candida albicans, a common source of yeast infections in humans.

STEP 5 – POSITIVE ACTIONS

- Try to include probiotics in your daily diet from food (ideally) or supplements – psyllium husk, slippery elm and Triphala.

- Take a spoonful of high-quality coconut oil for a minimum of three months.

- Make sure you are eating enough dietary fibre (prebiotics) through your food.

STEP 6

INFLAMMATORY LIFESTYLE ELEMENTS

◆———•●◆●•———◆

As you will now know from reading this book, what we put in and on our bodies represents the key to our health, including the health of our gut bacteria and the health of our intestinal lining. We all have a friend who eats junk food, drinks lots of alcohol and feels great and looks great. If you have psoriasis, this is not you. Sorry. Something has happened in your life to compromise your intestinal integrity and you can't get away with that flippant approach to food and lifestyle. Well, you can, but you will have to suffer the consequences.

For you (and me) elimination is an important and powerful part of healing your skin. I urge you to consider all the things that do not serve you; all the things that could be a barrier to your health; all the things keeping you sick; all the things keeping psoriasis in your life. Write a list right now of anything that could be having an impact on your skin. This could be anything from stress at work/in a relationship to smoking, drinking alcohol or eating highly processed inflammatory foods.

I have watched psoriasis wax and wane over 18 years. It is opportunistic – psoriasis thrives in a certain environment, and, consciously or subconsciously, you are creating an environment that psoriasis loves. Given the correct environment, things thrive. Think of your gut as a garden and change up the environment.

For me, the list was simple, but that doesn't mean eradicating these inflammatories was easy. Mindset and inspiration are key here! You need to want clear skin more than your current circumstances and potentially give up a few of your pleasures along the way. But, trust me, the benefits are worth it.

Inflammation can come from many sources, from emotional to pollution. Here is a list of the main ones:

Lifestyle inflammation

Smoking

Excessive alcohol

Drugs

Emotional inflammation

Negative self-talk

Destructive relationships

Anger/hate

Shame/embarrassment

Frustration/regret

Excess social media

Disempowering thoughts

Negative thoughts

Dietary inflammation

Sugar

Artificial trans fats

Refined carbohydrates

Excessive alcohol

Processed meat

Gluten

Dairy

For good reasons, people with psoriasis should also avoid:

- Junk food – anything high in salt, sugar or saturated fat (or anything deep fried)
- Nightshade vegetables:
    - Potatoes
    - Tomatoes
    - Eggplant
    - Peppers
    - Tobacco is also a nightshade
    - Goji berries!
- Pork
- Soya
- Peanuts
- Corn
- Eggs, in some cases – I ate eggs while healing psoriasis but not regularly

STEP 6 – POSITIVE ACTIONS

Some powerful steps in removing inflammation:

Lifestyle inflammation

- Write a list of why you want to stop.

- Replace bad habits with good habits.

- Join a support group/talk to your GP.

Emotional inflammation

- Connect with yourself – meditation, time out, deep breaths.

- Start neutral thinking. Neutral thinking is a powerful tool where you are less critical and judgemental and more balance.

- Gratitude journal – document three positive things each day (more if you can – I do ten).

- Put together a positive affirmation or mantra. This isn't for everyone, but I do this daily to focus me when day-to-day challenges zap my strength.

- Right now, be thankful for all the skin you have that is clear.

Dietary inflammation

- Focus on all the positive things you are eating and drinking.

- Replace inflammatory foods with green life-giving foods that support you gut bacteria and health.

- If you eat something on the inflammatory list, follow it up with lots of water or something cooling – for example, cucumber or celery.

STEP 7

ALCOHOL

◆———— • ● ◆ ● • ————◆

Alcohol and psoriasis do not mix. Alcohol is addictive, a depressant and a neurotoxin. Research into psoriasis and alcohol is overwhelming. If you have psoriasis, alcohol is a barrier to healing yourself. When I cleared my psoriasis, I stopped drinking for three months. I did actually start again and continue for a few years, so you can clear psoriasis and keep it clear while drinking, but I wouldn't recommend this. If you do decide to keep drinking, or drink after the three months, I would stick to clean spirits such as vodka and gin, and I would avoid beer at all costs, because of the gluten and yeast content

"Alcohol exposure can promote the growth of Gram-negative bacteria in the intestine which may result in accumulation of endotoxin. In addition, alcohol metabolism by Gram-negative bacteria and intestinal epithelial cells can result in accumulation of acetaldehyde, which in turn can increase intestinal permeability to endotoxin."
Alcohol and leaky gut

STEP 7 – POSITIVE ACTIONS

- Stop drinking alcohol for a minimum of three months, ideally a year.

- If you decide to drink again after this, try and reduce your drinking and only drink "clean" spirits with less sugar and yeast like vodka and gin.

STEP 8
MOVEMENT

◆———— • ● ◆ ● • ————◆

Move it or lose it! Movement and exercise are key to overcoming psoriasis as this will help you clear the build-up of toxins in the body and stimulate your sympathetic system, encouraging it to start healing.

In this review, _How lifestyle factors and their associated pathogenetic mechanisms impact psoriasis.,_ Madden et al. conclude that the data strongly suggests that improvements to disease severity can be made through dietary and lifestyle interventions, including increased physical activity. In the review entitled Lifestyle changes for treating psoriasis, it was noted that, for psoriasis, "… [a] combined dietary intervention and exercise programme probably improves psoriasis severity and BMI when compared with information only."

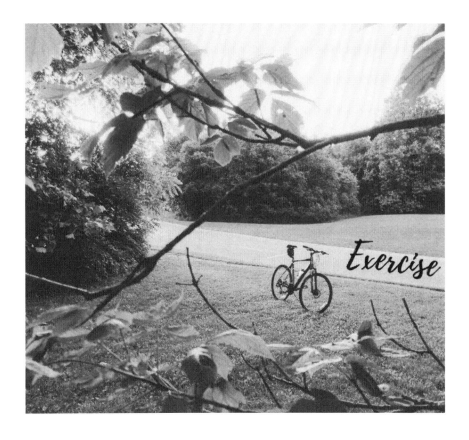

Sport and exercise for life

Sport is a great way to get fit. It helps us unwind, develop stronger bodies and gain better health. Team sports or social sports are particularly good. This can be tough at first if your skin is still bad – sport and exercise can bring a lot of anxiety relating to changing rooms/shorts and t-shirts etc.

STEP 8 – POSITIVE ACTIONS

I would recommend doing what you love and doing it often, such as walking, running or dancing – anything to get the heart pumping and the blood flowing.

Top tips:

- Make walking part of your daily routine – whether in the morning/at lunch or after dinner, just take 20 to 45 minutes out of your day to walk ... and relax. It takes 21 days to create a habit, and once a habit is in place it will come easily.

- Don't outsource your physical activity ⍰ – take the stairs, park the car far away from where you need to be or walk there.

- Look for forms of NEAT exercise.

- Do what you can, when you can. Try and find things that don't create barriers – do things at home with no equipment.

- Dancing is a fun way to exercise, so join a club or just dance about your living room – whatever you get involved in, get moving and get sweaty!

- Use YouTube – you don't have to sign up to anything new or get any equipment. There are about 3 trillion YouTube exercise videos online; everything from low impact to no impact – so what are you waiting for??

STEP 9
SLEEP

◆——— • ● ◆ ● • ——— ◆

Sleep is vital for healing but sometimes it can be challenging when you have psoriasis and you are itching a lot. I have so many memories of lying awake, itchy and in pain (often crying) and asking, "why me?". Unrelenting and aggravating itch feels like the worst form of torture. Sadly, in this life, many people live in terrible conditions or have bad experiences, but there is nothing quite so hellish as being trapped in your own body – your own personal and constant hell. It is for this very reason that I have written this book and why I wrote my first book, and also why I tweet more than anyone.

A lack of sleep is directly associated with psoriasis outbreaks as well as the deterioration of your general body condition, and a full night's sleep will help restore strength and help the elimination process.

STEP 9 – POSITIVE ACTIONS

- Plan to get a good night's sleep – between seven and eight hours.

- Exercise – regular exercise and physical activity will help you sleep.

- Prepare for sleep with:

  ◆ Relaxing baths

  ◆ Deep breathing

  ◆ Reading

  ◆ Wearing light, cotton clothes that don't make you itch

- Avoid alcohol, food and medication – these will keep you awake.

STEP 10

VITAMIN D

◆———— • ● ◆ ● • ————◆

Before I fully committed to diet and lifestyle intervention, I was in and out of remission with my skin, mainly because of vitamin D analogues or sun therapy abroad, so I really appreciate the importance of vitamin D in clearing psoriasis.

After my £3,000 trip to the Dead Sea, I started looking at cheaper alternatives and found Murcia – an inland salt lake in Spain with direct flights from Glasgow. Bonus.

I would go to Murcia twice a year for my skin, where I received short-term relief and had a relaxing holiday.

Each time my trip to Murcia would clear my skin and it would remain clear for three to six weeks when I returned. This was another short-term solution for me, and diet and lifestyle intervention remain the only things I've tried representing a long-term solution.

I now know that a number of things can impact vitamin D levels, including the health of your gut. According to Harvard Health, vitamin D that is consumed in food, or as a supplement, is absorbed in part of the small intestine. Various things can influence the level of absorption, including the integrity of the wall of the intestine (leaky gut) bile, stomach juices and pancreatic secretions. Consequently, conditions that impact the gut and digestion can reduce vitamin D absorption.

The active form of vitamin D, calcitriol, is considered more of a hormone than a vitamin and has the ability to activate over 1,000 genes in the body. Studies have shown that vitamin D deficiencies are associated with increased autoimmune development and increased susceptibility to infection from vitamin D and the immune system. This extract from a study on vitamin D and immunity highlights the importance of vitamin D in the immune response and the connection to the microbiome:

"There are plausible pathways whereby vitamin D deficiency can impair immune function, resulting in both overactivity and increased risk of autoimmune disease, as well as immune suppression with poorer resistance to infection. Vitamin D status may influence the bacterial flora that constitute the microbiome and affect immune function through this route. Exposure of the skin to ultraviolet radiation causes the production of a range of chemicals, including vitamin D, and new research is exploring possible vitamin D-independent immunomodulatory pathways."

More research needs to be undertaken in this area as this appears to be something that supports psoriasis sufferers topically through ointments, UVB and sun therapy.

This study, published last year, Dietary vitamin D, vitamin D receptor, and microbiome, states that "[a] Vitamin D supplement has a positive effect in IBD patients by modulating gut microbiome and also by increasing the abundance of potential beneficial bacterial strains"

In their diagram, they conclude that there are two main sources of vitamin D: exposure to sunlight and certain foods. However, I would argue that there is another way – through topical applications. According to the review, "Vitamin D and its receptor VDR regulate gut microbiome, maintaining barrier functions, and inhibit inflammation in [the] intestine."

STEP 10 – POSITIVE ACTIONS
• Get outside and expose yourself to safe sunshine daily when possible.
• Take a high-quality vitamin D supplement.

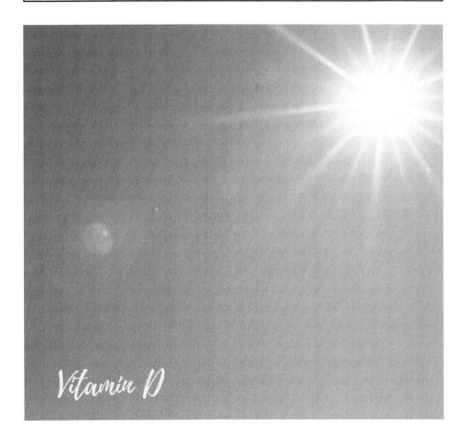

SUMMARY

◆————•●◆●•————◆

So, what do we now know? Here's a quick recap:

- Psoriasis has been newly classified as an NCD.

- It is believed that "NCDs are caused 'to a substantial degree' by tobacco usage, alcohol abuse, poor eating habits and physical inactivity".

- The cause of psoriasis remains unclear/unconfirmed, but we know there is an immune connection.

- All recent research leans towards disruption in gut microbiota (SIBO, dysbiosis) and leaky gut.

- Stress is an important factor in psoriasis and in gut microbiota.

- Gut bacteria impacts the skin and gut bacteria is disrupted in people with psoriasis, compared to controls.

- The abundance of the bacteria Akkermansia muciniphila is significantly reduced in patients with psoriasis. My abundance of Akkermansia muciniphila was significantly reduced when I had symptoms of psoriasis. My abundance of Akkermansia muciniphila was significantly increased when I was free from symptoms of psoriasis.

- Diet impacts gut bacteria significantly, especially prebiotics and potentially probiotics, and can maintain and repair gut lining.

- Vitamin D status can influence the bacterial flora that constitutes the microbiome and affect immune function on this route. Vitamin D regulates the gut microbiome, maintaining barrier functions, and inhibits inflammation in the intestine.

- Vitamin D supplements have a positive effect in modulating the gut microbiome and by increasing the abundance of potentially beneficial bacterial strains.

Lastly:

- ♦ There is a lack of robust research into complementary and alternative medicine/diet and lifestyle intervention for psoriasis. We need more good quality studies and we need them NOW.

- ♦ Thanks to the <u>Psoriasis Priority Setting Partnership</u> – this is now the No.1 priority for the Psoriasis Association –

- There is currently no official structure, advice or guidelines regarding complementary and alternative medicine or diet and lifestyle intervention for psoriasis. People rely entirely on Google and social media for guidance.

- In the UK we follow the NICE guidelines, which offer structure and guidance in relation to pharmaceutical intervention and UVB.

- The psoriasis pharmaceutical industry is set to be worth **$21.4 billion in 2022.**

IMPORTANT FINAL POINTS

- Psoriasis is multifaceted but I believe one thing causes they symptoms of psoriasis. I believe in cause and effect, one thing is the result of the other.

- I don't believe different things help different people with psoriasis. I believe there are a huge variety of things that can impact on the condition (along the disease pathway from symptom - root cause). Depending on the intervention, and it's position along the pathway, it will have short or long-term impact.

- Psoriasis waxes and wanes for a reason, there is a cause behind everything.

- I don't believe in 'spontaneous healing/remission'. People don't heal or go into remission spontaneously. Something changes, psychologically or physiologically, that impacts the cause of psoriasis or an element of the disease pathway.

- Diet and lifestyle intervention for psoriasis might not be an easy option but it targets the root cause and is the most powerful long-term solution.

Important points for you:

- If you do embark on diet and lifestyle intervention for psoriasis, your psoriasis may get worse before it gets better. It did for me and it has for many others. This seems to be a pattern and it is normal. This is outlined in Healing Psoriasis by Dr Pagano.

- STICK WITH IT. If you are really committed to healing your skin, stick with this for an absolute minimum of three months, ideally longer (perhaps six months).

- Don't beat yourself up. Don't beat yourself if you slip up or have a bad day or two. Talk kindly to yourself.

- Find solutions to manage your stress or, ideally, eradicate it.

- Ask for help and support (ideally from people who have read this book and know what they are taking about).

ABOUT THE AUTHOR

Lianne Campbell MSc is passionate about diet and lifestyle intervention for psoriasis and the emerging field of research into the human microbiome. After clearing psoriasis with diet and lifestyle changes after 18 years of being told diet would have no impact on her skin, Lianne became fascinated by the emerging developments relating to the human microbiome and focused much of her MSc in Digital Marketing on exploring, researching and sharing information online about the power of food and physical activity in treating skin conditions, and the important role the human microbiome plays in our health.

Lianne has a degree in Sports Management, an MSc in Digital Marketing and a diploma in Clinical Nutrition. Lianne worked for three years at a medical herbalist in Scotland called Napier's, where she learned a lot about diet, lifestyle and herbs. Following her sports degree, she went on to work for ten years in communications at **sport**scotland, the national agency for sport in Scotland.

On top of her academic qualifications, Lianne has over 190,000 hours' experience with psoriasis. She has woken up with psoriasis, spent the day with psoriasis and gone to bed with psoriasis every day since she was 16.

Website: www.fuelforhealth.co.uk

Twitter: @health_fuel

Instagram: @fuel_for_health

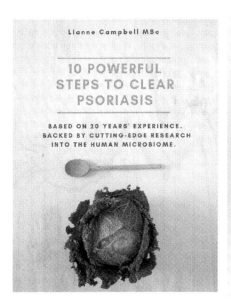

Lianne Campbell MSc

10 POWERFUL STEPS TO CLEAR PSORIASIS

BASED ON 20 YEARS' EXPERIENCE.
BACKED BY CUTTING-EDGE RESEARCH
INTO THE HUMAN MICROBIOME.

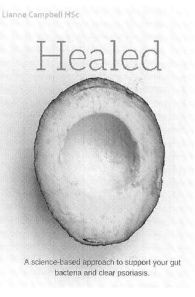

Lianne Campbell MSc

Healed

A science-based approach to support your gut bacteria and clear psoriasis.

Printed in Great Britain
by Amazon

58426304R00040